Early Beginnings

Early Beginnings:
Development in Children
Born Preterm

Barton MacArthur and *Anne Dezoete*

Auckland

OXFORD UNIVERSITY PRESS

Melbourne Oxford New York

Oxford University Press
Oxford University Press, Walton Street, Oxford OX2 6DP

OXFORD   NEW YORK   TORONTO
DELHI   BOMBAY   CALCUTTA   MADRAS   KARACHI
PETALING JAYA   SINGAPORE   HONG KONG   TOKYO
NAIROBI   DAR ES SALAAM   CAPE TOWN
MELBOURNE   AUCKLAND
and associated companies in
BERLIN   IBADAN

OXFORD is a trade mark of Oxford University Press

First published 1992
© Barton MacArthur and Anne Dezoete 1992
© Oxford University Press 1992

ISBN 0 19 558249 7

Cover designed by Chris O'Brien
Photoset in Sabon by Egan-Reid Ltd, Auckland
and printed in New Zealand
Published by Oxford University Press
1A Matai Road, Greenlane, Auckland 5, New Zealand

Contents

Preface

Early Beginnings: Development in Children Born Preterm evolved from a concern to help parents, families, and others interested in this very special group of children. It is hoped that increased knowledge will lead to greater confidence and more appropriate handling practices.

Initially, some basic definitions and explanations necessary for the understanding of this group and their treatment are provided.

In the section 'The Newborn Period', particular emphasis is placed on the needs of premature infants and the roles which they impose on parents.

The next stage, that of home-coming, brings with it another set of experiences for the family as they welcome the newcomer into the home and face patterns of feeding, sleeping, and crying which may be different to those generally expected of a young infant.

Frequently, questions asked by parents in the follow-up clinic are concerned with the mental, motor, and social development of infants. Sections have been included which deal with these concerns as they relate to infancy and preschool development. Discussion is based on research literature and twenty years of experience in a follow-up clinic with premature and other 'at risk' infants.

Next, the book presents what is probably one of the major problems in this area, and one that assumes greater importance as the years go by: do these children differ in school performance, or is there anything about preterm birth which delays school progress?

Caregivers are prey to many myths, and this book gives research perspectives for the long-term development of premature infants in their early years.

Case-studies written by parents provide valuable insights into the hazards of an 'early beginning' for the infant, and the difficulties experienced by the family. It can be seen that despite many initial obstacles, these children may have a positive long-term outcome and be a source of great pleasure to their families.

Finally, a theoretical section is included for readers interested in the topics of reciprocity, environment, and resilience, in relation to the field of preterm birth.

Barton MacArthur
Anne Dezoete

Acknowledgements

This book could not have been written without the many families who, over the years, have given us the opportunity to increase our knowledge of preterm infants and their subsequent development. We are especially grateful to the parents who provided photographs, and to those who shared their experiences in writing.

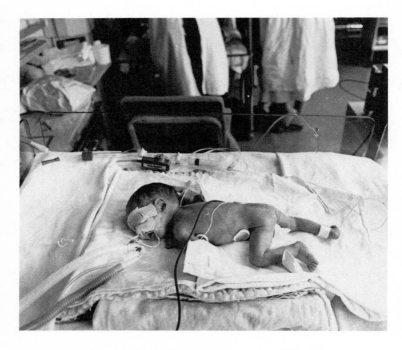

A newborn baby in an open incubator. *Innes Logan*

1
An Early Beginning

Introduction

This book has been written to support you as parents of a premature baby. When birth is premature or preterm (before the thirty-seventh week of pregnancy), it disrupts the normal course of events. It is natural, particularly for mothers, to feel angry and disappointed that this is happening to them. Often there is a period of grieving for the robust, bonny child that might have been.

To assist in understanding the confusing and seemingly unpredictable features of early birth and the subsequent development of the baby, we have set out some of the more common findings, and discussed practical issues of how to promote development and maintain positive family relationships.

Today, many premature babies are surviving who, a few years ago, would have died. This means that there are increasing numbers of immature infants with their unique needs that families have to cope with. In the United States of America alone, 250,000 families each year have this experience.

Definitions

During the time that your baby is cared for in hospital,

many medical terms will be used that need to be understood. If you do not grasp what a doctor or nurse is saying, ask them to explain what they mean. We have attempted to explain the more common terminology within the text.

The term 'low birthweight' (LBW) includes all infants weighing 2500 grams or less at birth, and 'very low birthweight' (VLBW) is employed most often when the weight is below 1500 grams.

Preterm infants may also be small for the number of weeks of pregnancy that have passed at the time the baby is born. These babies are called 'small for gestational age' (SGA) or 'small for dates' (SFD).

Incidence

Approximately five to seven per cent of all births in Western countries are under 2500 grams birthweight. Survival for many VLBW infants depends on specialized medical support. Currently this newborn care is represented by advanced technology in infant management, for example, methods of mechanical ventilation and feeding, together with an increased understanding of problems occurring around the time of birth.

New approaches in these areas continue to increase survival rates for VLBW infants, with those weighing over 1000 grams at birth almost routinely surviving, while infants weighing 500 to 1000 grams show a greatly improved outcome.

Causes

It is difficult to know the reasons for preterm delivery, due to the many complex factors operating during pregnancy. The cause of the majority of premature births is unknown. However, the following conditions have often been listed as contributing to prematurity:

1. Maternal complications during pregnancy (for example, diabetes, toxaemias of pregnancy, haemorrhage, infection, or disease)
2. Premature rupture of the amniotic sac (bag of waters) surrounding the developing foetus
3. Multiple pregnancy (twins, triplets)
4. Congenital malformation
5. A lower standard of living
6. Heavy smoking
7. Adolescent pregnancy

Mothers may worry that they have in some way contributed to the early birth of their baby. This should be discussed with the doctor, as the concerns are probably completely unfounded. Premature labour is not usually caused by activities such as healthy physical exercise, nor is it a punishment for past misdeeds.

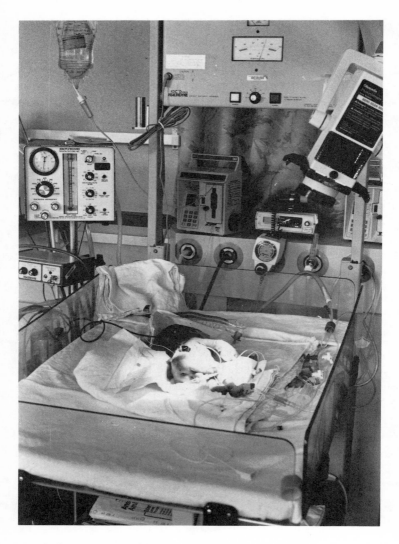

A baby surrounded by equipment in the neonatal intensive
care unit. *Innes Logan*

2
The Newborn Period

The State of the Infant

Because they are so immature, preterm infants often have difficulty with breathing, feeding, maintaining body temperature, and resisting infection. This means that they need to be placed in the protective environment of an intensive or special care unit.

Some infants are so ill that they must be connected to life support equipment. Because of this, parent–infant contact is restricted. For example, baby may be attached to a respirator (to assist breathing), and limbs may be immobilized for the administration of fluids to an artery or vein. Treatment with lights for jaundice (a common complication of prematurity) involves covering the eyes to protect them from the glare; this prevents baby from seeing for part of the day. Further, noise levels in the unit may interfere with the way baby processes sound.

Some of the problems associated with preterm infants are:

1. Immature lungs, which may lead to respiratory distress (difficulty with breathing)
2. Jaundice resulting from an excess of bilirubin (a yellowish substance produced when red blood cells break down)
3. Low resistance to infection
4. Feeding difficulties because the digestive tract is poorly developed, and sucking and swallowing reflexes are weak

5. Heat loss
6. Rupture of delicate blood vessels in the brain

A preterm baby may experience complications in varying degrees. Open communication between medical/nursing staff and parents is essential in order to increase understanding and relieve anxiety. Nurses and junior doctors generally keep parents informed of day-to-day events concerning their baby, and in most neonatal units it is possible to talk to the paediatrician who is responsible for each child. At times, crucial decisions about sick infants have to be made, and so it is important that you know and trust the staff. A doctor, psychologist or another trained professional will be available to help parents work through feelings of fear and grief at the impending loss of a baby who is given little chance of survival or of surviving without disability.

While there tend to be more long-term adverse effects for children of shorter gestation and lower birthweight (for example, less than 1000 grams), recent findings suggest that the majority of children studied, who are now between two and nine years old, are free of serious problems.

Prediction for the individual infant is difficult to make because of the tangled web of influences in the preterm child's development. However, it has been found that a good home background is a very important factor in outcome.

Role of the Parents

Even if the baby is relatively free from serious medical problems, parents of preterm infants often feel shocked and disappointed that the healthy baby they hoped for is instead a tiny, thin, fragile being whom they cannot hold, cuddle, or feed immediately after birth. As a mother, you may be angry that the baby was born early and blame yourself. Many mothers experience intense guilt.

For a number of parents, the birth of an infant long before the due date is a source of considerable grief. In some instances it may be compared with mourning for the loss of a baby. In fact, that is what it is — grieving for the loss of the full-term, 'normal' infant that was expected.

Some parents will go through recognizable stages of behaviour and emotions that are commonly associated with bereavement. At times there will be feelings of fear, anger, inadequacy, hopelessness, denial, and a variety of other emotional responses.

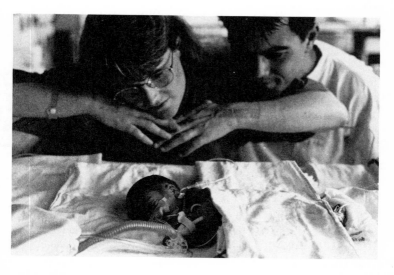

Parents visiting their baby a week after the birth. *Innes Logan*

One real fear is that news will be bad when parents telephone or visit the hospital.

Feelings of inadequacy at giving birth to, and subsequently looking after, such a small, delicate child, together with a sense of failure in the attempt at child bearing, may result in a lack of self-confidence.

Frequently there is sadness, as parents are aware of others taking home their full-term newborns after a few days. This may be further complicated by the uncertainty they sense in friends and relatives who do not know how to respond to this birth and the delay in the infant's home-coming. 'Normal' births and their celebration they understand, but how should they act when delivery is so premature?

If parents feel rebuffed by a preterm infant who does not respond in the way they had anticipated, or become frustrated by baby's 'atypical' behaviour, they may become somewhat detached in their attitude.

Sometimes, these anxieties and problems have a bearing on the later development of the child, for example, in the case of parents who continue to strive to help their child to 'catch up', even when development in preschool years is on a par with peers.

The extent or intensity of many emotions will vary according to the mother's previous history of childbearing, the support available from family and friends, and practical issues such as financial considerations.

Because the whole area of preterm birth is complex, parents should receive counselling in these early days to help them adjust to their new baby and to work through the phase of reconstructing their lives as smoothly as possible.

Mood changes can last for months after delivery, and

mothers have spoken of their extreme sensitivity to comments by hospital staff during the child's hospitalization. Indeed, the fact that infants are cared for by staff, sometimes for three or four months, may result in resentment and feelings of powerlessness on the part of parents.

Regular visiting can help increase your positive perceptions, and it has been found in at least one study that babies whose mothers visited most often were discharged from hospital earlier.

It is claimed that gentle stroking of the infant's head and limbs can result in increased weight gain, earlier release from hospital, and fewer complications. Fathers can participate in stimulating their infants through touch, and by providing tape-recordings of heartbeat, voice, and music.

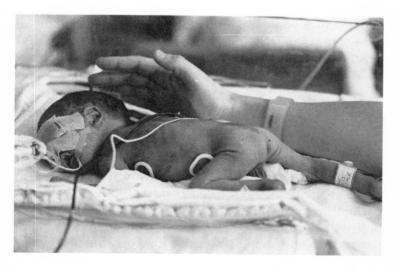

A mother stroking her baby. *Innes Logan*

19

Stimulation that comes too early, or is too much, is not helpful. Baby must be in an alert and contented state before she will benefit from enrichment.

Bold faces of animals and people, rather than pictures with lots of detail, appeal to infants and should be placed no closer than an average adult's handspan from the baby's eyes.

Cradled in a parent's arms at this distance, baby should be able to see the adult's face clearly. Closer and further away objects remain blurred (with full-term infants it is not until four months of age that they can focus as well as the average adult).

This ability to focus on an adult's face when held in a natural cuddling position, shows us that babies are ready for social responses from an early age. Watching your face, and listening as you smile and talk will help baby with later social, mental, and language development.

The more you can comfort and nurture your baby in the early weeks, the more he learns to relate to you as special people, and the more you can get to know your child.

Infant Nutrition

In the first weeks after birth, nutrition for the preterm infant is the decision of medical staff, and usually begins with intravenous fluids a short time after birth. When the baby is ready, oral feeding is commenced which, depending on the baby's condition, may be by breast, bottle, or naso-gastric tube (a small tube inserted through the nose to assist milk to reach the stomach). Mothers who had decided during pregnancy to breast-feed may feel that the choice was denied them with the complications of intravenous and tube feeding. However, neonatal intensive care unit staff encourage mothers to think about providing breast milk, as it is easier to digest, and it carries antibodies that protect the infant from infection.

From a mother's point of view, the most positive factors about breast-feeding are that:

1. It is something she alone can do for her child
2. It enables her to have bodily contact with the baby as soon as he is strong enough to suck at the breast

In order to establish and maintain lactation (production of breast milk) when a baby is small and sick and the mother is worried, a great deal of patience is needed with much support from husband, doctor, and nurses. The La Leche League (a national self-help group of nursing mothers), or a similar organization, can also provide assistance. Once full breast-feeding is implemented it is possible in many cases to continue indefinitely, and some mothers of preterm infants have reported successfully breast-feeding for eighteen months or longer.

Sometimes, despite every effort on the part of the mother, the attempt to breast-feed has to be abandoned. This should not cause you feelings of guilt — there are many reasons for difficulties with breast-feeding preterm infants related not only to factors within the baby, but to other influences beyond your control.

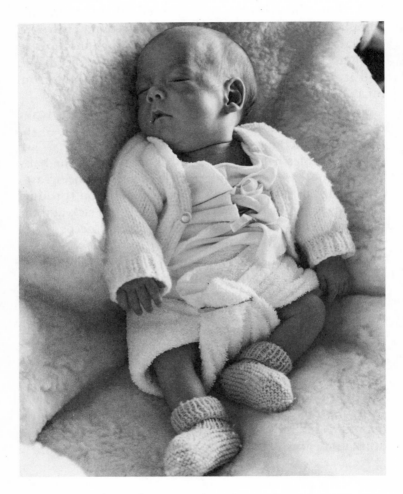

Home at last, after 2 months in hospital. *Innes Logan*

3
At Home

Homecoming

At last, after months in an intensive care environment, your premature infant is discharged from hospital. Many parents, especially solo caregivers, although happy at the thought of having baby to themselves, feel very nervous and vulnerable at this time. Caring for a baby around the clock is very different to visiting once or twice a day. As with any change, physical and mental preparation are necessary.

Some special care units have trained neonatal nurses who visit homes to provide support during the first few weeks after the infant has been discharged from hospital. Other public health services are available, but although many health professionals are used to larger babies, they are not necessarily experienced with small, preterm infants. It is therefore important for you to have names and contact phone numbers of staff who can assist with the more common problems associated with very premature babies.

Members of parent support groups can also provide information and encouragement, and many of these groups meet regularly to share experiences and knowledge. It has been reported that parents who participate in such groups tend to provide better care and feel more at ease with premature babies than parents who do not belong to self-help support systems.

The majority of preterm babies are discharged from hospital by forty weeks (term) or soon after. Parents tend to think that their infant is the same as a full-term baby, but generally the preterm child is immature in many areas, and not as 'organized' as a newborn full-term baby. Signals (usually crying) which baby makes to indicate needs such as hunger and tiredness may not be easy to interpret, and she may be unsettled, taking a long time to adjust to eating and sleeping routines.

The frequent feedings, crying, and night-time wakefulness can make parents exhausted. At this time it helps if you are well organized. An attempt to keep a routine and allow plenty of time to get ready for appointments and family outings should minimize stress.

It is also beneficial for the mother to become involved in something outside the home which is not related to infant care, even if it is only for a few hours a week to start with. This practice may assist later, when it is important for educational, social, and emotional purposes that mother and child separate, as for example, with school attendance. Because of the whole worrying upheaval around birth, you may not want to leave your child with other caregivers, and by the time he is three to four years of age there can be real problems with separation.

Feeding

Whereas in hospital decisions regarding infant feeding were made mainly by medical and nursing staff, now *you* are largely responsible for what and how to feed your baby.

If breast-feeding was going well before baby's discharge from hospital, support may be needed at home to keep your milk from drying up, as you become more involved in the busy schedule with your new baby. Sometimes breast-feeding does not work out in spite of adequate support and good intentions, and a change to bottle-feeding may be appropriate.

During the first year, cow's milk should be avoided. There are a variety of formulas which duplicate human milk as closely as possible, and are approved by doctors.

Because of their immaturity and the long period of intravenous and tube-feeding, many premature babies are slow to feed. Sucking may be weak and baby may tire easily, often falling asleep before enough milk has been taken. Usually baby makes up for this by waking and drinking more frequently.

If this becomes a problem and you consider that your child is not receiving enough nutrition, you should seek help from the doctor or health nurse. Weight gain in the early months is very important and this will be closely monitored.

In general, infants appear to gain weight and feed better when they 'demand' feed. However, when a baby decides its own feeding schedule, thought should be given to the parents' need for sleep at night.

It can be helpful in a two-parent family, where the infant is bottle-fed, for father to become involved with feeding. This not only gives mother a break, but enables father to spend time in close contact with his child. Feeding provides an opportunity for caressing, eye contact, and talking to baby, especially at this time when periods of sleep take up so much of the day.

Sleeping

The beginning of daily and nightly sleep rhythms is one of the most important of the developments in infancy, and when this has been achieved, family life is much more harmonious.

Sleep is, like food, an essential requirement for baby, and as with eating, problems may occur in early childhood. However, children differ in their sleep requirements — some appear to need a great deal of sleep while others sleep throughout the night but very little during the day.

It is nowhere more clear than in sleeping that families must adapt to the different style of development to be found in premature infants. For about six months after birth, premature infants generally sleep for longer periods but less regularly than full-term babies, and cry more when they are awake. This behaviour may affect the social development of preterm infants as it takes longer for parents to build up a relationship with their offspring.

The premature infant spends more time than the full-term infant in REM sleep, the sleep marked by rapid eye movements and fluctuations in the heart rate, blood pressure, and brain waves. (In adults, REM sleep is often called 'dream sleep'.)

At first, the premature infant may sleep more than sixteen to eighteen hours per day, with day and night mixed up. However, by nine months of age, most infants are sleeping through the night.

Research suggests many techniques to help soothe infants and achieve a sleep state, but finally, it is you who must, through watching and experimenting, work out the best method for your child.

Various techniques, including playing music, rocking, using pacifiers, singing to baby, and placing baby on a waterbed have been used to bring about sleep. Most forms of gentle rocking seem to calm babies.

Crying

Not only may premature infants cry more often than normal birthweight babies, but the crying may be higher in pitch. In fact, most adults have found the crying of a premature baby much more upsetting than that of the full-term baby. This may partly explain some of the handling problems parents have with premature infants. Further, during the first year, many parents have found that their preterm infants are not as easily pacified, and are more variable in mood than the infants of their friends and relatives.

There are several reasons why a baby cries. Crying may be caused by:

1. Hunger or cold
2. Pain
3. Overstimulation (that is, stimulation when baby is not in a relaxed and alert state)
4. Boredom or loneliness
5. Being undressed
6. The release of tension

Crying is the baby's way of letting you know his feelings or wants, of having a say in how things are organized. If you learn what your baby's cry means and respond to it, a feeling of trust will be built.

Mothers often ask about picking up their baby immediately and every time there is the sound of a cry. The question is really whether, if and when you respond quickly to the crying, baby will cry more often because she learns that it is a good way to demand attention, or whether the prompt response will eventually reduce the amount of crying.

Studies have shown that babies who at seven months of age cried more than other infants, have had mothers who were slower to respond to their infant's crying at three months of age.

You cannot spoil a very young baby; however there is no need to handle the baby at every little whimper. Normal development seems to require at least some crying.

There will be times when you think that nothing you do will console baby. Some mothers complain that their babies cry from about four in the afternoon until six in the evening each day, and no matter how much they try to soothe their baby, the crying continues.

If you are concerned that baby might be in pain or unwell, it is important for a doctor to examine baby. If he continues to cry a lot when there appears to be no physical reason for it, there may be times when you can place baby in a crib or bassinet and continue your work, or perhaps get someone else to relieve you for a short time. However, as with so many decisions, you must do what you are comfortable with — there are many individual differences. Some mothers feel much more at ease if they bathe, nurse with a rhythmic motion, or carry (in arms, front pack or sling) the crying baby. Others have recommended stroking and massage.

Remember, the amount or intensity of crying is not a measure of your worth as a mother. Crying is largely influenced by the baby's temperament, which in turn is shaped by many factors such as medical history, early experience, development, and inherited differences. Every baby has her own unique personality.

You will gradually learn to interpret cries, and the actual time your infant cries will reduce. This will also bring an increase in your own confidence and more opportunities for baby to learn from the home and the people in it.

Health

Preterm infants, especially those with chronic lung disease, are more likely to have respiratory infections within the first year or two after birth. Studies have found that around twenty to forty per cent of preterm infants who weighed less than 1500 grams at birth needed re-hospitalization within the first year of life. In contrast, the re-hospitalization rate for full-term infants is less than ten per cent.

Children cannot be protected from infection forever. Obviously they need to build up antibodies, but in the early months, it is wise for parents to take precautions with regard to visitors, and exclude those with infections from handling baby.

It is important to protect baby from environmental substances, such as cosmetic sprays and cigarette smoke, which may affect health. There has been much written about the dangers of 'passive smoking', and the hazards are even greater in the case of preterm children with their tendency to respiratory problems.

Doctors who are connected with the intensive care nursery, or your family physician, will examine baby at regular intervals during the first year. They will advise regarding immunization, but in general, unless there are contra-indications, the injections are given at the same age as for a full-term infant.

There is a two to ten per cent incidence of hearing loss among premature babies who weigh under 1500 grams at birth. Hearing checks are carried out by specialists within the first year and thereafter as considered necessary for each baby.

Visual difficulties (for example, with focusing) may also occur, particularly with the very small preterm infant. Eye examinations by an ophthalmologist are important, and your doctor will refer you to the appropriate person.

If you are concerned about your child's health, do not hesitate to seek medical attention. Early treatment usually leads to a more satisfactory long-term outcome.

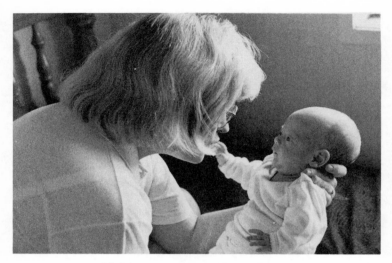

Making eye contact. *Innes Logan*

4
Development in Infancy

Factors Associated with Development

For ease of reference, mental, motor, and social development are discussed separately. In fact, these areas are inter-related, with skills in one very much depending on maturity or growth in others. There are several points which need to be taken into consideration when discussing development during the first two and a half years.

Firstly, development in infancy takes the form of a series of spurts followed by plateaux. While there is growth or progress in some areas (for example, motor skills involved in walking), there may be a temporary lull in other areas (for example, exploring objects using the hands and eyes).

Secondly, each baby is an individual, and development may depend on health, temperament and personality, everyday experiences, interaction with family members, and availability of services.

Thirdly, because of these differences between individuals, the average age at which children master tasks should be regarded as a range of months, not an exact point in time (for example, children are expected to first walk alone between ten and twenty-two months).

Fourthly, for years it has been debated whether or not, and how, the shorter period in the uterus should be taken into account when development is measured in early childhood. After all, a baby born following twenty-eight weeks in the womb, when examined on his first birthday, has been in existence for twelve weeks less than a full-term infant. Many developmentalists and doctors take this into consideration when looking at physical growth and milestones over the first two years.

Hospitals with large numbers of premature babies often run follow-up clinics where physical, mental, and motor development and behaviour can be monitored by experts. In most clinics, the reasons for carrying out these examinations are two-fold: for the individual baby and family to detect and remedy any problems as early as possible, and to provide a long-term evaluation of the newborn services.

Mental Development

When we talk about the mental or cognitive development of infants and children we are interested in how well they find, sort, and use information. It is something which goes on developing, but at different rates for different children, as each child learns from her environment.

In their everyday world there are many ways for children to have experiences which will aid cognitive development. For young children these may include activities such as discovery, finding what things mean, and sorting and remembering information. As children grow older these will include testing ideas, making decisions, solving problems, understanding rules, and thinking ahead.

During the first year of life infants learn a great deal about the way the world operates — much more than experts in the past realized. If they are retained in hospital for long periods there will be less opportunity for gaining this sort of experience and, when considering cognitive development, it may be necessary to take this into account.

One well-known American researcher said that as a group, very low birthweight infants did not have even mild problems in sixty per cent of cases. Other studies have reported, in infancy, severe handicap in anything from five to eighteen per cent of these children.

Detailed studies have found some VLBW children to be slower in the development of eye-hand co-ordination and visual perception. This may have influenced their performance in some of the cognitive areas.

Often parents ask how they can help with the mental development of their infants. There are a number of ways that you can assist, and at the same time gain a great deal of enjoyment.

Here are a few examples for premature children of various age groups (these are approximate only — children develop at different rates).

Four to eight months:
- Talk to baby
- Show interest and enthusiasm for baby's own sounds
- Introduce new sounds and words
- Sing nursery rhymes
- Play with soft, squeaky toys and rattles
- String beads or animals in front of baby to promote reaching

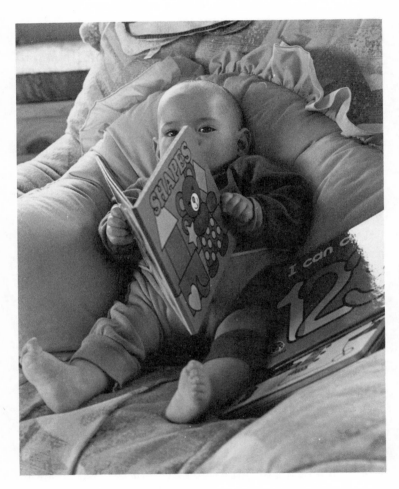

Ben (1340g, 31 weeks gestation), aged 8 months. *Innes Logan*

- Give baby opportunities to explore objects placed in her hands

Eight to twelve months:
- Play games (for example, pat-a-cake, peek-a-boo)
- Imitate baby's activities (for example, banging blocks together)
- Help baby to search for hidden toys under cloths, upturned cups or boxes
- Look at picture books
- Sing rhymes
- Repeat early words, such as mama, dada, nana, baba

Twelve to eighteen months:
- Hide objects (seek and find)
- Point to pictures in books, make animal noises
- Repeat names of everyday objects
- Give simple instructions (for example, put the spoon on the plate, cup on the table, toys in the cupboard)
- Place blocks into containers
- Fit shapes into holes
- Play with mechanical toys (an adult should be present)
- Promote self-help activities as a game (for example, eating with a spoon and dish, dressing)
- Demonstrate relationships by play acting (for example, making a doll stand, sit, lie, hugging a doll, brushing hair; placing a cup on a saucer, drinking from a cup)

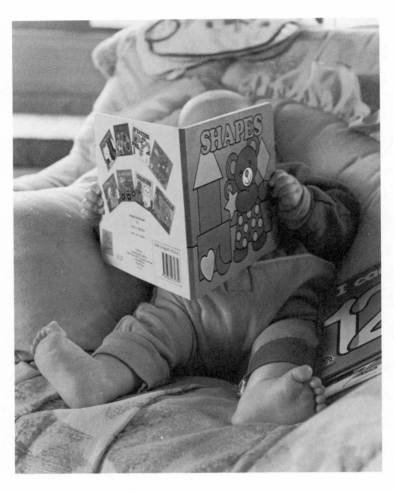

Ben, reading, aged 8 months. *Innes Logan*

Eighteen to thirty months:
- Hide and find objects behind furniture
- Play hide and seek games with other children/adults
- Roll, throw, kick a ball
- Put things together in sequence (for example, feeding a doll, putting it to bed, dressing and undressing it)
- Build with blocks
- Place shapes in holes
- Play with mechanical toys
- Play repetitive word games
- Read stories, tell stories about the family, go to the library to choose books
- Draw with crayons

Speech and Language

Language is a system of communication from one human to another. It is very much related to general development, environment, and maturation of the nerves and muscles.

Receptive language (understanding what is said) usually comes before expressive language (the ability to use words to describe and explain). Parents frequently say that although their child is not speaking, he can understand and carry out simple instructions.

Expressive language is often slower to develop in premature infants. Research evidence suggests that fifteen to thirty-five per cent of VLBW infants have delayed speech and language skills at two years of age. However, as with mental development, there is extreme variability between children, with some having few recognizable words around two years of age, while others may combine words into long sentences by this age.

It is important to pick up delays in receptive and expressive language because of their later influence on development and behaviour. A child who cannot understand, or make himself understood, becomes upset, taking out the frustration on himself, caregivers, siblings, and peers. It is better to intervene before such behaviour starts.

In infancy, your child's language skills should progress from non-verbal communication (for example, smiling in response to your smile), to early vocalization (cooing with pleasure, growling with displeasure). This is followed by the imitation of sounds, from those known to new ones. Later comes babbling, gesturing, and responding to his own name and to simple requests.

By approximately two and a half years of age your child should have an intelligible vocabulary of at least fifty to one hundred words, and be able to join words together in simple sentences, point to pictures in a book, and name common objects.

It has been found that language learning is helped by joint attention during interaction between the child and the caregiver — that is, by making sure baby is looking at you when you speak, that the radio is not blaring, and that you remain alert to the child and listen for a response. It is not helpful for parents to talk non-stop to baby — she needs time to practise and experiment with what is heard.

Books which contain simple, bright, bold illustrations can be introduced as soon as baby shows an interest

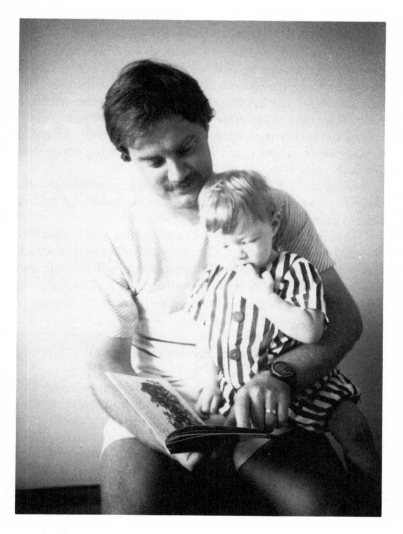

Michael (1035g, 28 weeks gestation), aged 18 months.

(usually at around six months of age). With very active babies, looking at pictures while sitting on an adult's lap will capture attention and slow down the activity level. Initially, baby may be interested for only a few minutes but, with your enthusiasm as you talk about the pictures, point to them and act them out, baby will concentrate for longer periods. It is better to have a short session several times a day promoting language in this way, than to expect your infant to sit for twenty minutes while you work through a whole book.

You will find that through everyday interaction with baby, certain key words are repeated again and again. This is essential for language learning.

Listening to nursery rhymes and jingles with repetitive words appeals to babies. Good tapes are available which can act as an ideal camouflage for the not too tuneful adult voice. You may be surprised at how early your child begins to try to sing along with familiar tunes.

Motor Development

Gross motor skills involve the use of large muscles, such as those concerned with rolling, sitting, and walking. Fine motor skills involve the use of small muscle groups, as in grasping and manipulating objects with the hands.

Muscle strength and control improves during infancy. Early movements are large and jerky but gradually become smoother and more purposeful.

It is well known that VLBW children tend to be slower in motor development than their normal birthweight age-mates over the first two years or so. Often premature infants are slower to sit alone, crawl, and walk unaided. Parents frequently expect their children to walk soon after they start cruising around furniture, but many do this for months before gaining the balance and confidence to start to walk alone. When the muscular system is ready, the majority of children will attain the necessary competence.

However, if you suspect that your baby's limbs are floppy or stiff, or that he is too slow in reaching motor milestones, you should seek advice from your doctor. A number of extremely premature infants with motor delay are referred to specially-trained paediatric therapists to promote motor development.

Parents can encourage motor skills in the following ways:

Gross Motor:
- Spread a blanket on the floor so that baby can practise lifting the head, raising the chest (press-up position), rolling over (encourage this by placing a toy nearby), and crawling
- Place cushions on the floor to support baby in a sitting position until she is strong enough to sit unsupported
- When baby shows signs of wanting to stand and step, encourage her to pull herself to standing position by placing colourful objects on top of a low, sturdy table or armchair
- Help support baby when she attempts to walk — walking with adult support usually precedes walking alone
- At around eighteen to twenty months climbing onto chairs is a popular activity

Fine Motor:
- Hands are often clenched during the first months — encourage baby to open them by stroking the palm and giving baby a rattle to hold
- Place your young baby in a semi-upright position to assist him to move his hands towards suspended objects
- Hang safe, brightly coloured mobiles within reach so that baby can bat at and reach out for them
- Place objects nearby that make an interesting noise when banged together
- At around nine months of age, introduce container play, for example, blocks dropped into and tipped out of boxes
- Provide soft toys with interesting faces for baby to explore
- Wooden blocks are ideal for stacking one on the other
- At twelve to eighteen months encourage baby to feed himself with a spoon and to drink from a cup — don't worry about the mess
- A favourite game at around eighteen months is scribbling with crayons on newsprint
- At eighteen to thirty months, children like to sit on their own chair at a small table. Pouring and filling activities with sand and water appeal to this age group

Growth

After the first few months of special care and with

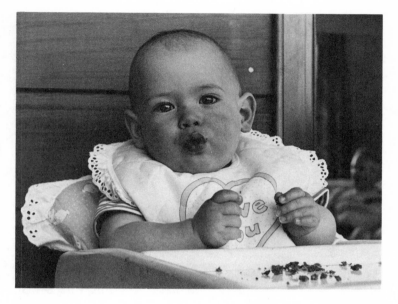

Ben using his fingers to feed himself at 1 year. *Innes Logan*

adequate nutrition, physical growth rate usually accelerates. Some babies catch up very quickly, while smaller and more sickly infants often take longer to achieve their growth potential.

Many babies who weighed under 1000 grams at birth (particularly those who were small for gestational age) remain small and underweight during infancy and childhood.

If you consider that baby's growth is not progressing as it should, seek professional help during your routine attendance at clinics held by your doctor or health nurse. You will also be advised about infant feeding — which

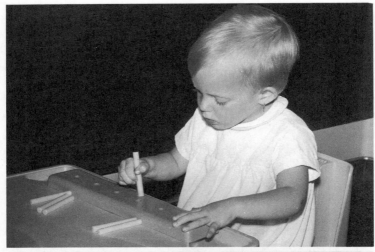

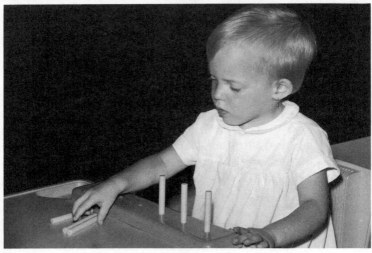

Krystal (690g, 29 weeks gestation), at 2 years 5 months, fitting rods into holes.

milk formula to use if you are not breast-feeding, and when to introduce solids.

Social and Emotional Development

From birth, babies display emotions that have a number of uses. Through them, infants are able to 'tell' us about their moods and feelings, as well as to control those around them by the way they respond to people and form relationships.

At the same time, infants are coming to recognize emotions in other people. All of this helps them with a lesson which began in the first few months of life. They are learning that they are a 'self', separate from others. Between themselves and the world, this independence becomes a very important influence on behaviour as time goes on.

One of the first social acts that an infant displays is smiling. He becomes increasingly careful as to who will be favoured with a smile. The growth of smiling shows us how the child is developing socially.

Another behaviour which we observe early is attachment. This is a form of social relationship, where the infant seeks to be with certain people. It is a relationship where love is given and returned.

Later social behaviour is strongly influenced by relationships in the first year, and usually those infants who are securely attached become the most well adjusted socially.

Many parents of premature infants say that they are

'very active and strong-willed'. In one study, measures of temperament and behaviour of one hundred VLBW infants in the first ten months after birth revealed that the majority were rated by their mothers as medium (compared with high and low) in activity level. Most were fairly regular with biological functions (such as feeding and bowel motions), positive in mood, and showed an approach (rather than withdrawal) response to new things around them. Eleven per cent were rated by mothers as more difficult than average in temperament/behaviour, which was approximately twice the percentage for full-term infants of similar age.

Clinically, it has been found that some children who are highly active become less restless as they grow older and are guided by their parents. A few need professional intervention to help them settle.

A child who is described in infancy as 'very determined' may be considered 'stubborn' throughout life, or, it may be a passing phase as he learns to cope with feelings of anger and frustration.

With independent mobility, and the discovery of so many new experiences, the two-year-old is working out that she is a unique person, different from mum and dad, and there is a need to try out limits.

This can be a time of testing for parents, but you need only continue the disciplining you started with baby soon after home-coming. Discipline is not punishment, it is helping your child to understand what behaviour is expected of him as a member of your family, and of society.

Some children are more difficult to discipline than others because of their individual personality. These children may need more love and attention, and are more of a challenge than an 'easy' child.

Decide with your partner what behaviour is important to encourage or discourage and be consistent in your demands. Do not fuss over every little incident. Try to anticipate situations which may lead to unacceptable behaviour. These may be when the child is bored (unoccupied during hours of conversation between adults), tired (social event continuing past the child's bedtime) or subjected to inappropriate stimulation (visiting shops with attractive displays of delicate, expensive articles).

A child who has been guided wisely (without physical punishment) is more likely to trust, to have self-esteem, and to believe that she has an important part to play in successful relationships within the family.

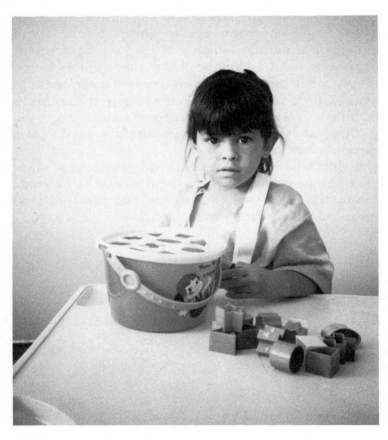

Shanice (700g, 24 weeks gestation), aged 3 years.

5
Preschool Performance

Except for size, by approximately two and a half to three years of age, most children who were born prematurely are not able to be distinguished from their full-term peers. Allowance for the period born preterm is no longer as significant when looking at development, and counts for only a few points in developmental tests.

In general, parents who have spent the first two years worrying about their child's health, report that he is no longer prone to illness, and sleeps and eats well.

Development forges ahead during this period. Language proceeds very rapidly, with the four-year-old enthusiastically telling stories about events at preschool. Creative play increases as more use is made of imagination. Self-help skills are enhanced with importance placed on toilet training and emphasis on greater independence in dressing and eating.

Speech and Language

As speech is learned, not instinctive, children need to be exposed to the speech of others. Language input must be geared to your child's level of development, not so simple that she remains unextended, and not so complex that it is beyond her understanding.

Language is learned firstly in the family, through interaction with parents, older brothers and sisters, aunts, uncles, and grandparents. Reading and talking to your child, patiently listening to his attempts with new words, describing how objects work, playing, and taking him on outings helps this learning. When watching television, you may like to view the programme with your child, explaining various points of interest, and singing or acting along with those on the screen.

As mentioned earlier, when considering development, the 'normal' range is wide. From three to five years of age, language skills which are expected to develop include:

1. Using four- to six-word sentences about the actions of others, for example, 'Mummy is talking to Nana'
2. Singing or saying rhymes or television jingles
3. Relating everyday happenings to caregivers
4. Correctly answering simple questions such as, 'Where are you going?', 'What are you eating?'
5. Asking more and more questions
6. Requesting help when trying difficult tasks
7. Using verbs (action words) and changing common words into plurals

Because a large number of premature children have early language delay, if you think your child is not speaking clearly or using language in a similar way to others of the same age, check with the preschool teacher, psychologist or doctor. Referral to a speech/language therapist may be necessary. Progress is usually steady and most children who have had problems earlier make themselves clearly understood by school age.

Cognitive Skills

Studies from many parts of the world conclude that the premature preschool child is one who must be followed closely because of the number whose development is slower than or different in pattern to other children.

However, when looking at this information, it is important to take into account the child's birthweight. For example, some studies show that infants weighing less than 1000 grams have more long-term delays (including slightly slower mental development), tend to be smaller in size, and have more difficulties after school entry, than larger babies.

A number of these outcomes may not be detected until past infancy or at school age. A child may seem to be progressing satisfactorily at one and two years of age, only to show discrepancies in areas of learning at three or four; or a four-year-old who has an overall ability score within the average range may have some kind of learning disability later.

A good home environment and stimulating everyday experiences are known to be associated with better outcome, and the majority of children who were born prematurely grow up to lead normal lives.

Preschool organizations can help with activities that are not easy to provide at home, but there are many games which are fun for you and your child and which help to prepare for the school years.

Three years of age:
- Drawing: first circles, then squares and faces — point out these shapes in pictures

- Puzzles: simple activities involving fitting or sorting circles and squares; grouping things according to shape or colour — human faces or bold, bright puzzles of animals are suitable
- Stories: while looking at books, provide plenty of opportunity for children to explain pictures that are not too detailed; at the same time encourage them to tell their own stories about recent experiences (for example, going for a ride in a train, helping grandmother at the supermarket)
- Comparisons: use objects such as sticks, buttons or blocks to give plenty of practice in comparing things (for example, bigger/smaller, more/less, long/short)
- Colours: there will be many chances to talk about colours in all of these 'games'. Pay particular attention to naming and matching objects that are red, yellow, or blue
- Counting: at this stage counting should be practised out loud using actual objects, for example, 'Count these blocks', 'Give me two buttons'. (Don't put a lot of pressure on your three-year-old and be pleased if he can count accurately to two or three)

Four years of age:
- Drawing: continue with circles, squares, and copying straight lines; talk about triangles. This is also a good opportunity to encourage left to right move-ment, which is important for later reading and printing
- Puzzles: from grouping involving circles and squares to finding particular shapes that have been mixed in with others

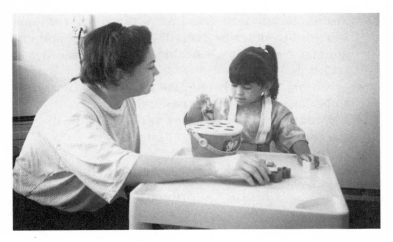

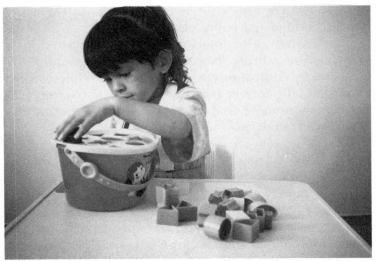

Shanice, aged 3 years, working with shapes.

- Stories: talk about stories and pictures. Ask the four-year-old to describe everyday happenings and encourage her to talk about things in the same order in which they happened
- Counting: gradually increase the number of objects to be counted; move on at the child's pace
- Comparisons: use pictures and objects to discuss 'tallest', 'smallest', 'biggest', 'same'

Motor Co-ordination

By the time your preschool child reaches five years of age, he should have very similar motor skills to the other children at kindergarten or playcentre.

Fine motor co-ordination, so important for later printing and writing, is maturing, and your child will show better control of crayons or pencils while holding them using the correct grasp. Drawings and paintings are thought about more, and several shapes and letters can be reproduced at this age.

Book pages are turned one at a time, and beads threaded on a string are proudly presented to mum as a necklace. Buildings are erected from blocks, and water in a cup is carefully carried without being spilled.

Improving gross motor co-ordination is apparent in everything your preschooler attempts. Stairs, ladders, trees, and playground equipment are climbed with increasing confidence. Running and jumping are included in play, and she is able to move around any obstacle that is in the way. Ball games are popular, with kicking, throwing, and catching a large ball starting to be within her capability. Pedalling a tricycle provides hours of amusement.

During the preschool period your child learns to become more independent. Self-help skills improve, and he is able to eat a meal without assistance, manage zippers or large buttons, put on and take off a jacket, brush teeth, wash and dry hands, and use the toilet (complete bladder and bowel control should be achieved before school entry).

Some children have difficulties in motor areas and may need assistance or special therapy to meet these goals. They may be very cautious when trying anything new, and extra patience and encouragement is needed to build confidence.

As parents, it is important that you provide lots of opportunities for your child to practise motor skills, so that she may feel the same as other children of the same age, and is as ready as possible to meet the demands of school. There are a number of preschool gymnastic groups operating which are very enjoyable and increase confidence. It is best to observe for a session before enrolling, to check whether supervision is adequate and that you will be getting value for money.

Social Maturity

From clinical experience, it is evident that during the preschool years a number of children who were premature are rather immature in self-help areas and socialization.

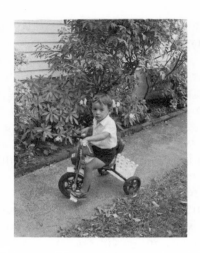

Jacob (890g, 28 weeks gestation), aged 3 years.

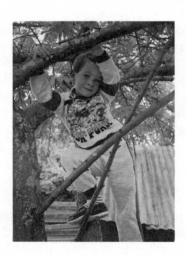

Jacob, aged 4 years.

Sometimes, because it is quicker and less messy to help young children with feeding, toileting, and dressing, rather than letting them do it themselves, they may not get the chance to practise self-help skills. At times, children are 'not ready' to advance in these areas, and are slower than their peers despite parental encouragement.

It is important to support your child in his growth towards independence. By school age, most children can:

1. Take off and put on a coat, dress or shorts unassisted
2. Button (large) or zip up a coat
3. Eat with a fork and attempt to use a knife for spreading
4. Get a drink and food unassisted
5. Wash and dry face and hands
6. Care for themselves at toilet, and go through the day free of accidents (night accidents may occur rarely)
7. Avoid a variety of hazards (for example, are aware of the possibility of a dangerous fall, do not play with matches or broken glass, keep off the road, and are watchful when crossing roads)
8. Help with simple household tasks
9. Amuse themselves well in play
10. Play co-operatively at preschool level
11. Play games involving simple rules (for example, hide-and-seek, tag)
12. 'Perform' (sing, dance) for others

If your child is having difficulties with self-help and socialization, remain positive. Most children respond well to praise, and aim to please.

Parents who belong to support groups may be offered advice and given pamphlets on how to handle minor problems, but if your child does not appear to be progressing in certain areas (for example, bladder and bowel control, getting along with age-mates) your doctor can refer you to a psychologist who commonly deals with these aspects of learning.

Expectations

It is recognized that problems of any kind are handled more effectively when people are sensibly confident, and believe that they can play an important part in influencing what happens in their lives or the lives of their families.

Over and over again, those working with infants and children who were born prematurely have found that difficulties with adults' expectations concerning the development of these children are at the base of the problems. So often this is an outcome of the baby's early days when she was small, frail, less responsive, slow to feed and, in general, different to other infants of the same age.

This difference may give rise to fears which result in over-caution and lack of stimulation on the part of parents or other family members who have been deeply affected by the condition of the infant at birth. On the other hand, parents and others may be over-demanding and unrealistic. They may be anxious that the child should 'catch up' as soon as possible. This is particularly so during the preschool years when parents become more aware of any delays and the effects that these may have on school progress.

All family members (including siblings and grandparents), need to understand that each premature child had a unique beginning, and continues to be a unique individual whom they may help to achieve the best possible quality of life.

Do not attempt to push your child's development before his nervous system is ready. If you do so, it will make you and your child very frustrated.

Follow a middle course as far as stimulation is concerned. If you feel stressed, if the child is unwilling, fearful or shows signs of fatigue, if eye contact is more difficult than usual, or if activities are not giving you both enjoyment, then consider whether what you are doing is appropriate. When you are conscious of the need for the right amount of stimulation you will soon become sensitive to your child's signals.

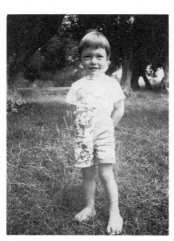

Jeremy (750g, 25 weeks gestation), aged 3 years.

Give your child love, guidance, and the chance to have many new experiences. A warm, relaxed approach to promoting development (whether it is walking or toilet training) brings the best results, with the child progressing at her own pace, encouraged by your support.

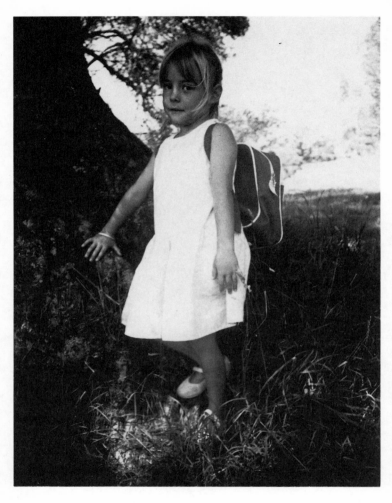

Going to school. Adele (925g, 25 weeks gestation), aged 6
years.

6
Starting School

Learning and Behaviour

Whilst the vast majority of preterm infants have intelligence test scores that are within the normal range for the population, a number have problems that interfere with school work.

Much still has to be found out about the pattern of strengths and weaknesses displayed by premature children on various measures of mental development. There is some evidence that in the early school years they may have difficulties with copying shapes and letters, and with other tasks involving visual motor integration.

Children who were preterm often do less well than their full-term peers at tasks where they must respond to something they have heard or seen, particularly if they have to be assessed through a different sensory area, for example, writing answers to material they have listened to. Some premature children have unusual score patterns when they are tested, rather than overall low scores on intelligence tests.

Having said this, it should be emphasized that research has demonstrated many times the importance of the home environment. The family plays a large part in influencing what happens, and whether problems that occur can be eliminated or made less through positive experiences.

It would seem that the family influence is much more important for the development of premature infants than it is for full-term infants.

Recently, some developmental psychologists have noted that very small premature infants, at school age, often display behaviour problems in the classroom. As infants they were easily distracted and very active. This behaviour continued into school years to the displeasure of their teachers, who were probably unaware of the background of these pupils. Much more research needs to be done before we will be able to predict which premature children will cope well with school and which will not.

Unfortunately, developmental problems are not always easily detected before school years. This is made even more complex by the manner in which young children may find ways to make up for or to hide these developmental differences. It is often only at school age, when the child is placed in more demanding situations, that these delays or difficulties become obvious.

When considering this information, it must not be forgotten that premature children are all individuals, not just one group of children with the same features. They come with contrasting temperaments, many different backgrounds (both medical and home), and a great variety of rates and patterns of development.

The following are some suggestions which may help your school-age child:

- Always make time to talk to your child about school as a new and interesting experience. *Listen* to what he says about the school day
- Keep in touch with teachers; be aware of what your child is doing at school; be positive and keep things in perspective; take a sensible approach to teachers — you both have the same goal — the well-being and progress of your child

- Continue to share stories, and to read and talk about books — this may continue to teenage years and is a wonderful way to learn and to enrich a relationship. Initially, listen to and discuss a sentence or two each day, but avoid becoming a 'teacher'. Make your child feel confident about and interested in reading
- Many ex-prems are still physically small when they enter school. In some instances this may need special handling, but these children must not be 'babied' — they resent this and it delays their development
- Some children will require assistance with self-help skills (toileting, washing hands, and taking off and putting on clothes) early in their school life. As mentioned previously, often children who were preterm are immature in these areas, and this can lead to frustration for both teacher and child. A little thought with appropriate clothing and training can make undressing and dressing easier for activities such as swimming
- In social skills or mixing with other children, your child may be resistant, sensitive, and inclined still to cling to you. If this is happening, ask the advice of the teacher, but above all think about your own feelings and behaviour and be decisive — perhaps the child senses your own anxiety and reluctance to part with her
- Sometimes motor skills are slow in developing. This is another area where practice can be fun — throw and catch beanbags and balls, encourage balancing on low walls, beams, and outdoor playground equipment

In these beginning school years the aim should be to

make your child realistically self-confident. At times you may be hesitant about asking for advice or help. Don't be timid about pressing for discussion with a professional. There are some things which your child may not be 'outgrowing', and the sooner remedial assistance is provided, the better.

Finally, parents viewing their children happily participating in school activities often voice the fears held around birth, and say how thankful they are that such immature, sick infants have turned out to be little different, or no different, from other children of the same age (refer to the case studies of Leonie and Michaela, Ruth, DJ, and Kylie).

7
Summary

The lonely and dramatic event of preterm birth makes parents of these children part of a very special group, with a growing membership in many countries.

In the majority of cases prematurity has no known cause.

Whether or not the preterm infant experiences complications during hospitalization, communication between parents and staff, and parental contributions to the well-being of the baby through frequent contact and later feeding practices, are important in the development of family relationships.

Because of their fragility, premature infants have problems that are unique to their immature state. Parents are often shocked and disappointed at the birth of a tiny baby, and require the support of friends and professionals at this time.

On discharge there is a great change in the organization of family life as parents take over the care of their premature baby. Caring for baby gives parents many opportunities, not only to get to know their infant but also to assist with his development. Support groups are available to help with behaviour and health.

Each baby is an individual, and development may depend upon personality, everyday experiences, interaction with family members, health, and availability of services.

There appear to be certain features of behaviour which are more common in premature infants in the preschool period, and there is much that parents can do to assist development and preparation for school.

A number of children who were born preterm do have problems with some aspects of school work, but research has shown the importance of a good home environment in reducing these.

8

Case Studies

Leonie and Michaela — Our Miracle Babies

At twenty-two weeks gestation I was diagnosed as carrying twins (a scan at sixteen weeks had shown only one baby!). One of the babies was surrounded by an abnormally large amount of amniotic fluid (polyhydramnios). Because it continued to build up I was admitted to hospital to prevent premature labour. However, at twenty-five weeks the bag burst, and Leonie (who had been the baby with excess fluid) was born, weighing 700 grams (1lb 9oz); her twin sister Michaela followed at a mere 510 grams (1lb 2oz).

The meagre size of the babies was a shock to everyone, but they were in good condition, which gave us all hope. I had been given two series of steroids beforehand which helped the babies' lungs immensely in those crucial early days. Michaela's kidneys didn't function for the first two days, but finally she had her first 'pee' and all in the Unit were jubilant! During the early weeks the twins experienced the usual conditions of such prematurity. Leonie had extra problems when the catheter in the umbilical artery had to be replaced by one inserted through an

artery at the top of her right leg. Unfortunately, a block-
age occurred, causing her to lose circulation to the leg and
toes, and resulting in her leg turning black. We were told
that she would lose the leg, but after several days of the
leg being in an oxygenated bag, circulation returned.

Meanwhile, Michaela battled on remarkably to the
amazement of her doctors, having fewer problems than
her 'big' sister. She was a real wriggler and had to wear
mittens to stop her from pulling out her tubes. She lay on
a special mattress filled with water to help reduce stress,
and appeared to love this waterbed.

Continual attempts over three months to breast-feed
the babies were unsuccessful, but I continued to express
milk for the twins until they were five months old.

We were fortunate living in a small city as the hospital
was so close to our home, enabling us to spend a
considerable amount of time at the Unit. Life was hectic,
as at home there was an eleven-month-old, a five-year-
old, and a seven-year-old requiring my care. But I had a
very caring husband as well, and supportive friends who
eased my load considerably.

The twins came home three and a half months after
their birth, and all went smoothly for the first few weeks,
when they developed feeding problems and failed to
thrive. After tube feeding them ourselves at home for
several weeks their weights picked up and they gradually
returned to sucking properly. The reflux they had both
developed, slowly improved with age. Apart from this and
constant ear and chest infections, the first year at home
was surprisingly uneventful.

At eighteen months of age, Michaela is a normal,
energetic little girl learning to take her first steps. Leonie

has moderate cerebral palsy and still has problems with her right leg, but is otherwise a bright and happy child.

To our knowledge, Leonie and Michaela are two of the smallest surviving twins, and we consider ourselves to be very fortunate.

Ruth

As the tiny, wide-eyed, pink bundle of humanity was wheeled past in the incubator towards the Neonatal Intensive Care Unit, I recovered from our daughter's birth, soberly taking stock of what was before us. Five years before, our first daughter had been born eleven weeks early at 1550 grams. Now our second daughter, Ruth, had arrived fifteen weeks early, a mere 870 grams (1lb 14oz). I knew that before us lay a long haul of disappointments, joys, setbacks, milestones, hopes, and a requirement of stoical patience and endurance.

As a mother of a very premature infant, I needed space to work through my grief — grief for the healthy, plump, independent full-term baby I had hoped to deliver. Over the ensuing weeks I repeated the cycle of grief several times — disbelief, anger, depression, and finally acceptance. Painful triggers assailed me constantly — the sight of a woman blooming in late pregnancy, friends' babies who were thriving, alert, and robust, and the contrasting spectre of our own child subjected to unpleasant and unnatural interventions amid a daunting array of probes and tubes monitoring her every breath.

For the initial weeks Ruth's chances of survival were paramount in our minds. Once assured of her survival and that her future would not be compromised by her prematurity, we allowed ourselves the luxury of thinking ahead. We moved from being apprehensive spectators at the Unit to becoming involved participants in Ruth's care — touching and cuddling her, supplying expressed breast milk, and informing ourselves more confidently and accurately about her progress. There became a security in the routine of visiting twice daily and in familiarity with the ward routine.

Ruth's dependency within the Unit was mirrored by our own emotional and social dependence on friends and family. We learned to receive meals, babysitters, phone calls, gifts, and mail — appreciating unconditional support when we knew we could not reciprocate. At many points our faith in God alone kept us buoyant as the long weeks stretched on. It was essential to take one day at a time.

Ruth was discharged at fifteen weeks of age, on the date she had been due. The tiny bundle of skin and bones was now a healthy, rounded, contented baby whose 'premature' tag was soon to fade. Today she is a normal, healthy three-and-a-half-year-old who interacts happily and actively with our other three children. While the trauma surrounding her birth is already a retreating memory, we have a special appreciation for her life, and special empathy for those who are coping with a premature birth in their family.

DJ

As we watched DJ hop properly and determinedly at a recent sports day, we felt not only proud of our son but also relieved that our five-year-old was doing all the things the rest of his peers were doing. DJ was born twelve weeks premature, weighing just over 1200 grams (2lb 10oz), and had many of the problems associated with babies of that weight and gestation.

By the time a term baby is six months old, parents can usually see where their child's development is at, and can look forward to watching their child grow and develop like other children. It has taken us nearly five years to achieve the feeling of 'he's going to make it'. As parents, we found it difficult not knowing the what, when, why, and how of developmental milestones. Although DJ would achieve steps, he never did them at the times stated in the textbooks.

He had strengths, such as being a very early talker, which he used to advantage. Often he would talk his way out of doing an activity which he didn't like or couldn't do. DJ did present with some of the problems mentioned in the literature. For example, he had perceptual difficulties. He would love to go to the local park, but trying to get him to slide or swing resulted in a screaming episode if his feet left the ground. From early days we had help from the visiting developmental therapist who assisted us to direct his activities so that he could achieve. Sometimes it seemed to be a ticking off of each skill mastered, and as the skills grew so did his confidence and self-esteem. He began setting his own challenges — for example, recently he taught himself to ride a scooter. He practised and practised, and when he succeeded he came running in and said, 'Quick, come and look, I can do magic'. It was a great moment.

When we think back on some of the frustrations and challenges we experienced during those early years, such as teaching him how to play, to separate from us, and to use the toilet, it seems so long ago now. Today he is a happy, healthy boy who brings us great joy and pleasure.

Kylie

It all started when I went to the doctor for my regular monthly checkup at 23 weeks. I was pregnant with twins, so had been taking it easy and felt really well. The doctor had other news for me. My blood pressure was high and I had protein in my urine. He told me I had to go straight to the hospital for bed rest. Once there I had a scan and was told that the twins were very small and did not have much chance of survival unless I could get to 28 weeks gestation. Scans during that time showed that both babies were growing but one baby was not growing as well as he should be. At 27 weeks a test showed that the bigger baby was under

stress, so an emergency caesarean was
performed.

The first delivered was our little girl Kylie, weighing
605 grams, and then our little boy Tony weighing 280
grams. Tony only survived 20 minutes and all effort was
put into ensuring Kylie would live.

Kylie's first week in the Intensive Care Unit went with
no hiccups and at two days of age we were able to hold
her. Then at one week, she had her first distended tummy.
She was taken off her one millilitre of breast milk every
four hours and put onto antibiotics. Then her patent
ductus needed to be closed with medicine. This channel
was to open two more times but was closed successfully
after the last course of indomethacin.

Difficulty with accessibility to veins to insert the vital
drips was causing problems, so a central line was inserted
under general anaesthetic. However, this line came out
and a second one had to be put in. While having this
procedure she suffered a cardiac arrest. Fortunately, she
was resuscitated easily but afterwards she became very
sick. Her oxygen requirements went up, she became
oedematous and was very susceptible to handling. It was
all touch and go for a few days. Suddenly she came right,
and after six weeks of being ventilated she was able to go
on to CPAP and eventually head-box oxygen.

At this time I had been expressing four hourly during
the day so that she would be fed breast milk through her
feeding tube, and in the hope that she would be able to
breast-feed in the future. However, when the time came to
suck, Kylie found it hard work. She went back to
requiring oxygen when feeding. Bottles were started with

the aim of encouraging her to suck. I became down-hearted and gave up expressing after four months.

Eventually, after five months in hospital, Kylie came home. She still required oxygen during feeding and was on a special milk formula. We used special teats with bigger holes cut in them so that she did not have to exert herself so much with sucking. We also had an apnoea mattress which would sound an alarm if Kylie stopped breathing.

Our time in the Neonatal Unit was not easy. It was very stressful and difficult. There would be days when things would be going okay, then bang, we would take several steps backwards. It was an emotional roller-coaster. We also had the stresses of everyday life to cope with, while fitting in as much time as we could at the hospital and still trying to ensure a happy environment for our two-year-old son, Jason.

Our experience was helped by the dedication of the paediatricians, nurses, and all the other staff involved in the Unit. They were always there to talk and to listen. We could ask to see them or ring at any time. Many of them were part of our support crew.

Now here we are two years on. We have just celebrated Kylie's second birthday. She is a normal, happy, cheeky, loving little girl. Last week she started climbing out of her cot, and we have had to buy her a bed. There followed a week of chasing her in and out of the bedroom. Her determination is amazing, but now we have finally won!

9

Some Theories

This section has been included to assist any readers who would like some direction in continuing their reading of research and theories from the field of preterm birth, and for groups seeking topics for discussion.

Introduction

The search for evidence concerning the consequences of low birthweight owes a considerable debt for its early impetus to the workers who studied cerebral palsy.

Joerg in 1828 has been quoted as saying: 'Too early and unripe born foetuses may present a state of weakness and stiffness in the muscles persisting until puberty and later!' (Little, 1853).

In their comprehensive review of the latter years of the eighteenth century and the early years of the nineteenth century, Wallich and Fruhinsholz (1911) wrote:

> It is indeed a responsibility which one assumes with
> reference to another human being in imposing upon him a
> premature birth. One must before interrupting a
> pregnancy when the life of the mother isn't exposed to an
> immediate risk be very well warned, all things being
> otherwise normal, of the physical and intellectual values,
> actual and in the future, or the social value of the product
> obtained.

In this quotation there is evidence that by early this century some familiar questions about the future of those born prematurely were being asked, during a controversy which arose from the debate concerning therapeutically-induced premature delivery.

Over the years which followed to the beginning of the Second World War the field was marked by the contradictory nature of the data and conclusions (Benton, 1940). Discrepancies arose because of, among other reasons, methods of assessing cognitive development and biased methods of sample selection.

One of the major problems with the early research was the failure to take into account both gestation and birthweight. Gruenwald (1965) stated that the baby whose weight was not appropriate for his gestational age was quite different in prenatal and postnatal characteristics when compared with infants who were low birthweight and preterm.

This was a watershed in low birthweight research, as up to this point most findings were based on the conventional cut-off point of 2500 grams and below or under 2500 grams; therefore, the population studied included a mixture of low birthweight infants of both full and short term.

Over the last two decades the growing technical complexity of neonatal intensive care units has been associated with a significant increase in survival rates for VLBW infants (Kilbride et al., 1990). As Cooke (1991) writes: 'There have been many reports describing improvement of survival of preterm infants over the last twenty years'. This increased survival rate has given rise to many issues that have a bearing on the quality of life of preterm infants.

The question as to whether the techniques that keep increasingly more immature babies alive result in an increase in infants with an abnormal outcome is seen by some as a benefit confounded by the risk of developmental problems (Carran et al., 1989). Views of this nature are in keeping with the concept of 'failure of success'.

Prematurity is associated with many variables, and it is not possible to separate it from the many events with which it is associated (Oberklaid et al., 1991).

When one considers the influences that are present in the life of a preterm infant — hospitalization, separation, and fragility to name a few — it becomes obvious that there is unlikely to be a one-to-one relationship between prematurity and outcome. For example, if we consider school performance of low birthweight infants, there are many factors that determine differences including social class, minor neurologic dysfunction, and psychological variables modified by neonatal illness, family separation, and long-term hospital stay.

In past years research in many follow-up studies sought to demonstrate a relationship between reproductive complications and abnormality. For some, this concept came to be referred to as the 'continuum of reproductive casualty' (Pasamanick and Knoblock, 1966). Advocates of this approach to research are concerned with a variety of reproductive conditions and their associated outcomes for the child, ranging from the subtle, which may be so imperceptible that they cannot be measured successfully by known methods, to abnormalities of a marked and serious nature.

The contemporary view is that a single risk factor such as prematurity is insufficient when studying outcome or making predictions. We cannot, for example, ignore the environment provided by the family. This may represent states from minor discord to serious disruption. The term 'continuum of caretaking casualty' (Sameroff and Chandler, 1975) has been coined to represent this influence.

For the most reliable results in prediction both of these views must be included and the transactions between the 'continuum of reproductive casualty' and the 'continuum of caretaking casualty' considered (Hetherington and Parke, 1986).

Reciprocity

Traditionally the infant was seen as a passive being, shaped by environmental forces. However, a number of people have recognized the active role played by the infant.

It appears from the statements of researchers that infants take some control even before birth. Nearly thirty years ago, Liley (1967) presented the concept of a foetus as being 'in a very large measure in charge of his environment'. The findings of Liggins (1969) also served to emphasize the part played by the foetus in initiating the onset of labour. Increasingly, developmentalists are coming to appreciate that the behaviour of infants is not only complicated, but that it also has an influence on those around them.

This suggests that the infant is a complex organism with an individual pattern of reactivity and activity — a pattern that will affect the interests of parents. Active characteristics and styles of behaviour displayed by the infant will assist in initiating the caretaking behaviour of the parents.

Hsiu-Zu Ho (1987) concluded that we are uncertain as to whether a positive caregiving environment accelerates development or whether the more advanced infant elicits more responses from the mother.

It seems likely that the behaviours are reciprocal, and that the infant is simply reinforcing the parents' behaviour. Thus the behaviour of the caregiver helps to release and determine the infant's responses whilst the infant's response also shapes the parents' behaviour. This has been referred to by developmentalists as reciprocal determinism (Bandura, 1985). Through the transactional model (Sameroff and Chandler, 1975) a method is available to describe the long-term bi-directional or reciprocal relationships with particular reference to the social and economic context.

From birth this reciprocity is reflected in all those behaviours and characteristics of the infant which help to determine the stimulation that he or she receives. Note that characteristics are included as well as behaviour. The infant's physical characteristics release a number of responses on the part of the mother, for example, eye contact or physical contact. The parents also tend to respond to infant behaviour in the same mode — where there is vocal behaviour the response is likely to be vocal (Osofsky, 1979).

Conversely, when handling the infant, there are physical characteristics which may cause the mother to respond in a more negative manner. The infant's muscle tone may affect the way that the mother handles the baby. Furthermore, it is possible that this and other physical characteristics will influence her own emotions and cause her to feel rejected or depressed.

At first it is difficult to think of the newborn as a social being, but newborns who are within the normal range for development are equipped with a number of behaviours which attract parents, or other adults for that matter, and ensure that their attention is held. Although there are not many of these behaviours, those that are available are very useful in gaining attention and interest. Good examples of this are crying and smiling. When the infant ceases crying when attended to or smiles in response to a smile, the caregivers' behaviour is being reinforced. We must also remember that this process is bi-directional, and that the adult has distinctive features, such as a voice, which interest the infant.

Bee (1989), when considering these reciprocal behaviours, suggests that, from birth, the parent and the infant are 'programmed' to join in a 'crucial social dance'. This forms the basis of the developing relationship which will be crucial so far as the development of the parents' attitude to the child is concerned.

These distinctive qualities and responses in a normal baby are an important element in reciprocal behaviour, and this is one of the reasons why parenting is easier for predictable and happy babies (Vander Zanden, 1989). However, the traits of low birthweight babies often do not fall within this normal range of behaviour, and then may not be conducive to the establishment of reciprocity described above, and in some instances their behaviour may be beyond the experience and coping skills of the parents.

Als and Brazelton (1981), in a study of preterm infants, found that these infants were less responsive and more disorganized in all their interactions than were the full-term infants. Further, these authors noted that while on the one hand the preterm infants were less likely to respond, the parents on the other hand were increasing their attempts to obtain a response, and were less likely to establish a 'dialogue' with their infants than the parents of full-term infants.

In his consideration of 'interactional deficits', Minde (1984) contends that premature infants demonstrate these deficits early in life and that they appear to be independent of other medical complications. He links these interactional deficits with the crisis which the parents of these infants pass through that may leave them depressed and may compromise later parent-child relationships.

In a rather paradoxical way there is some hope to be found here. If problems were solely the result of any physiologic insult during the perinatal period then there would be little that could be done. However, many parents succeed very well with these children. It is important that we should learn from them, provide emotional support for those who require it, and ensure that the opportunities exist for those who wish to learn adequate parenting skills.

Environment

Through the transactional model (Sameroff, 1986) it is possible to study the reciprocal or bi-directional effects of parents and infants within a particular social and economic environment.

In the transactional model of child development,

outcomes are considered in the context of the transaction between the child's behaviour and the context in which it is observed.

Among theories which may be applied to the understanding of environmental variables as they influence the development of a child is that of Bronfenbrenner (1980). In this theory there is a reciprocal interaction between, in this instance, the infant and the environment. For Bronfenbrenner the environment is not just the immediate home setting but also the connections with wider environments. The infant's removal from the hospital and placement in a family is an ecological transition, and Bronfenbrenner would argue that this ecological transition is not only a consequence of, but also an initiator of developmental processes.

Much has been written about the environment either linking low socio-economic status with low birthweight (Richards, 1982), or with the outcomes of that condition (Leonard, 1990). For example, a study by Klein et al. (1985) found that school performance may be influenced by lower socio-economic status in very low birthweight populations.

Investigations of this nature have made it clear that to predict outcome both the 'biologic risk' and the quality of the environment must be considered (Bauchner et al., 1988).

Research indicates that the socio-economic status of low birthweight infants is possibly a marker for potential psychological risk factors leading to developmental and behavioural morbidity.

Whatever the environment, an interesting topic for developmental psychologists is the transition to the new environment when the caretaking role is undertaken fully by the parents or parent. There may be responsibilities in the care of the VLBW infant which are greater than had been anticipated by the parents. Apprehension for any family may result from unusual caretaking demands (Beckman, 1983), the grieving process accompanying the birth of a VLBW infant, fears about the infant's vulnerability (Affleck et al., 1986), the appearance of the baby (Perehudoff, 1990), or the lack of confidence or loss of the 'ideal' child, to name but a few.

When parents become responsible for the care of an infant with less than the expected competence, the potential for problems in the interactive process is high (English et al., 1988).

Resilience

Finally, the question which many developmental psychologists are asking now is why children with similar backgrounds and histories differ in developmental outcome. Why are some children resilient so far as the influences of risk in infancy are concerned whilst others are seemingly vulnerable to them?

Though there is comment and conjecture about this phenomenon there is little research. A number of studies contain groups of low birthweight infants who could be regarded as vulnerable because of their early history, yet when assessed as school children show no evidence of delayed development (Sameroff and Chandler, 1975).

Why does this happen? Is it because there are self-righting influences at work that enable the child to 'catch up' if they are in a satisfactory environment? Some would also consider that low birthweight infants have recourse to alternative pathways that permit them to continue in their progress towards developmental goals.

Whatever the influences and their outcomes, the researcher in the field of low birthweight soon becomes aware of the multiple risk factors that may operate to slow development and cause delay in cognitive growth. There appears to be evidence here to support the 'cumulative stress hypothesis'.

Clearly, in any study of vulnerability and resilience the model of development which is applied will make a great deal of difference to the conclusion. If the model is a mechanistic one then development is viewed as:

> . . . a linear chain of invariant causes and invariant effects . . . early traumas are linked to subsequent sympto-matology and predictive inefficiency is viewed as a result of some failure to locate the critical links in the chain of causation . . . (Sameroff and Chandler, 1975: 189)

Unfortunately, prediction of outcome in terms of cognitive functioning from birth to infancy or preschool and school-age years has not been as reliable as both researchers and clinicians would consider desirable for their decisions.

In the study of resilience there is hope that a contribution may be made to the improvement of the reliability of prediction if studies are designed to obtain information concerning infants who were at risk yet did not display atypical development (O'Grady and Metz, 1987). These are the false positive children who present developmentalists with a number of challenging questions.

Low birthweight studies have much to contribute to the study of resilience, as they have been described as 'major contributors to the "vulnerable child" syndrome' (Bachner et al., 1988).

The terms 'resilience' and 'vulnerable' have been used in the above comment, but other terms have also been employed, and the children have been described as 'invulnerable' (Garmezy, 1981) and 'stress-resistant' (Antonovsky, 1979).

O'Grady and Metz (1987: 5-6) adopted the following definition of resilience for their study:

> . . . an unusual or marked capacity to recover from or cope successfully with significant stresses, of internal and external origin.

In this study the authors examined psychological adjustment of children aged six or seven years for its relationship to infancy risk status. They concluded that the interactions which were obtained demonstrated that life events 'magnify synergistically' the adverse effects associated with these risk factors but that social support and internal control orientation may reduce the effects of stress.

In another interesting study, Werner and Smith (1982) examined a group of children with a history of family instability and perinatal stress or low birthweight. The resilient children in this group differed from their peers in that they were more likely to be first-borns, had easier temperaments as infants, more social support, fewer stressful life events, and had developed an internal locus of control orientation by adolescence.

The implications of studies such as these for low

birthweight infants are considerable. The trends of these findings indicate that there are some clear directions for intervention with these children. There appear to be strong arguments for developing and extending support systems for them as well as seeking ways in which to develop locus of control with an internal orientation.

Four centuries ago Shakespeare turned his attention to the topic that we have addressed here when he provided us with a description of the outcome of preterm birth for one of his characters. Let us finish on a positive note and give Shakespeare the final word:

> . . . on her frights and griefs,
> Which never tender lady hath borne greater,
> She is something before her time deliver'd.
> . . . A daughter, and a goodly babe,
> Lusty and like to live: the queen receives
> Much comfort in't . . .
> (Emilia, in *The Winter's Tale*, Act II,
>   Scene 2)

References

Affleck, G., Tennen, H., Allen, D.A. and Gersham, K. (1986) Perceived Support and Maternal Adaptation During the Transition from Hospital to Home Care of High-risk Infants *Infant Mental Health Journal* 7 (1).

Als, H. and Brazelton, T.B. (1981) A New Model for Assessing Behavioral Organization in Preterm and Full-term Infants. Two Case Studies *Journal of the American Academy of Child Psychiatry* 20: 239-63.

Antonovsky, A. (1979) Health, Stress and Coping *New Perspectives on Mental and Physical Well-being* San Francisco, Jossey Bass.

Bandura, A. (1985) A model of Causality in Social Learning Theory. In Mahoney, M. and Freedman, A. (eds) *Cognition and Therapy* New York, Plenum.

Bauchner, H., Brown, E. and Peskin, J. (1988) Premature Graduates of the Newborn Intensive Care Unit: A Guide to Followup *The Pediatric Clinics of North America* 35 (6): 265–72.

Beckman, P. (1983) Influence of Selected Child Characteristics on Stress in Families of Handicapped Infants *American Journal of Mental Deficiency* 88: 150-6.

Bell, R.Q. (1968) A Reinterpretation of the Direction of Effects in Studies of Socialization *Psychological Review* 75: 81-95.

Bee, H. (1989) *The Developing Child* New York, Harper and Row.

Benton, A.L. (1940) Mental Development of Prematurely Born Children; Critical Review of the Literature *American Journal of Orthopsychiatry* 10: 719-46.

Bronfenbrenner, U. (1980) *The Ecology of Human Development: Experiments by Nature and Design* London, Harvard University Press.

Carran, D.T., Scott, K.G., Shaw, K. and Beydouin, S. (1989) The Relative Risk of Educational Handicaps in Two Birth Cohorts of Normal and Low Birthweight Disadvantaged Children *Topics in Early Childhood Special Education* 9 (1).

Cooke, R.W.I. (1991) Trends in Preterm Survival and Incidence of Cerebral Haemorrhage 1980-9 *Archives of Disease in Childhood* 66: 403-7.

Crnic, K.A., Greenberg, M.T., Ragozin, A.S., Robinson, N.M. and Basham, R.B. (1983) Effects of Stress and Social Support on

Mothers of Premature and Full-term Infants *Child Development* 54: 209-17.

English, B.J., Parry, T.S. and Donovan, M. (1988) Early Behaviour, Development and Parenting in a Very Low Birthweight Infant Group *Australian Pediatrics* 24: 25-9.

Escalona, S. (1984) Social and Other Environmental Influences on the Cognitive and Personality Development of Low Birthweight Infants *American Journal of Mental Deficiency* 88: 508-12.

Garmezy, N. (1981) Children Under Stress: Perspectives on Antecedents and Correlates of Vulnerability and Resistance to Psychopathology. In Rakin, S. (ed) *Further Explorations in Personality* New York, Wiley.

Gruenwald, P. (1965) Some Aspects of Foetal Distress. In Dawkins, M. and MacGregor, W.G. (eds) *Gestational Age, Size and Maturity* London, Spastics Society, Medical Education and Information Unit.

Hetherington, E.M. and Parke, R.D. (1986) *Child Psychology: A Contemporary Viewpoint* McGraw-Hill, New York.

Ho, H.-Z. (1987) Interaction of Early Caregiving Environment and Infant Development Status in Predicting Subsequent Cognitive Performance *British Journal of Developmental Psychology* 5: 191.

Kilbride, H.W., Daily, D.K., Claflin, K., Hall, R.T., Maulik, D. and Grundy, H.O. (1990) Improved Survival and Neurodevelopmental Outcome for Infants Less than 801 grams Birthweight *American Journal of Perinatology* 7: 160-5.

Klein, N., Hack, N., Gallagher, J. and Fanaroff, A.A. (1985) Preschool Performance of Children with Normal Intelligence who were Very Low-Birth-Weight Infants *Pediatrics* 75 (3): 531-7.

Leonard, C.H., Clyman, R.I., Piecuch, R.E., Juster, R.P., Ballard, R.A. and Behle, M.B. (1990) Effect of Medical and Social Risk Factors on Outcome of Prematurity and Very Low Birth Weight *Journal of Pediatrics* 116: 620-6.

Liggins, G.C. (1969) Fetus in Control. In Wolstenholme, G.E. and O'Connor (eds) *Ciba Symposium Fetal Autonomy* Churchill.

Liley, A.W. (1967) *The Fetus in Control of his Environment* Montgomery Spenser Memorial Oration, RACP.

Little, W.T. (1853) *On Deformities* London, Longmans.

Minde, K.K. (1984) The Impact of Prematurity on the Later Behavior of Children and on their Families *Clinics in Perinatology* 11 (1): 227-44.

Oberklaid, F., Sewell, J., Sanson, A. and Prior, M. (1991) Temperament and Behavior of Preterm Infants: A Six-year Followup *Pediatrics* 87 (6): 854-61.

References

O'Grady, D. and Metz, J.R. (1987) Resilience in Children at High Risk for Psychological Disorder *Journal of Pediatric Psychology* 12 (1): 3–23.

Osofsky, J. (1979) *Handbook of Infant Development* New York, Wiley.

Pasamanick, B. and Knoblock, H. (1966) Retrospective Studies on the Epidemiology of Reproductive Casualty: Old and New *Merrill-Palmer Quarterly of Behavior and Development* 12: 7-26.

Perehudoff, B. (1990) Parents' Perceptions of Environmental Stressors in the Special Care Nursery *Neonatal Network* 9 (2) 39-44.

Richards, M.P.M. (1982) Low Birthweight Infants — Family Repercussions *British Journal of Hospital Medicine* November 480-3.

Rutter, M. (1979) Protective Factors in Children's Responses to Stress and Disadvantage. In Kent, M.W. and Rolf, I.I. (eds) *Primary Prevention of Psychopathology* Hanover, NH, University Press of New England.

Sameroff, A.J. and Chandler, M.J. (1975) Reproductive Risk and the Continuum of Caretaking Casualty. In Horowitz, F.D. (ed) *Review of Child Development Research* 4, Chicago University Press.

Sameroff, A.J. and Seifer, R. (1983) Familial Risk and Child Competence *Child Development* 54: 1254-68.

Sameroff, A.J. (1986) The Social Context of Development. In Eisenberg, N. (ed) *Contemporary Topics in Developmental Psychology,* New York, Wiley, 273-91.

Thomas, A. and Chess, S. (1977) *Temperament and Development* New York, Brunner/Mazel.

Vander Zanden, J.W. (1989) *Human Development* New York, Alfred K. Knopf.

Wallich, V. and Fruhinsholz, A. (1911) Avenir Éloigné du Prématuré *J. Am. de gynéc. et d'obstet.* Par 2 VIII: 625-55.

Werner, E.E. and Smith, R.S. (1982) *Vulnerable but Invincible: A Study of Resilient Children* San Francisco, McGraw-Hill.

Zarling, C.L., Hirsch, B.J., and Landry, S. (1988) Maternal Social Networks and Mother–Infant Interactions in Full-term and Very Low Birthweight, Pre-term Infants *Child Development* 59 (1): 178-85.

Glossary

Amniotic fluid   Liquid in which the foetus floats. It provides protection against injury and temperature changes

Anoxia   Lack of sufficient oxygen in the brain

Antibodies   Proteins produced by the body to deal with harmful substances in the bloodstream

Apnoea   Cessation of breathing. Apnoeic attacks are episodes, often recurrent, in which breathing is interrupted

Apnoea mattress   A machine that sounds an alarm to warn staff/ parents that there is a pause in baby's breathing

Birthweight
- Low birthweight (LBW) A baby weighing less than 2500 grams (five and a half pounds) at birth
- Very low birthweight (VLBW) A baby weighing less than 1500 grams at birth
- Extremely low birthweight (ELBW) A baby weighing less than 1000 grams at birth

Cardiac arrest   Sudden stoppage of effective heart action

Catheter   A tube, usually made of plastic, used for infusions or to drain fluid

Cerebral palsy   A non-specific diagnosis given to children with some impairment of muscle tone, movement, and co-ordination

Cognitive development   Growth of mental activities such as remembering, thinking, learning, and perceiving

Contra-indication   Indication against the use of a particular substance or treatment

CPAP   (Continuous positive airway pressure) delivery to a baby who is breathing spontaneously, of a flow of air/oxygen under slightly raised pressure. Used to assist a baby's breathing and to reduce the frequency of apnoeic attacks

Developmental psychologist   A psychologist with particular interest in the stages of growth and development

Distended abdomen   Abdomen swollen by pressure from within (stomach, bowel)

Foetus   The unborn baby from the eighth week of gestation until birth

Gestation   Length of the pregnancy at the time the baby is born

Head-box (oxygen)   A box placed over a baby's head to provide extra oxygen

Glossary

Hypoxia   Lack of oxygen
Incubator   A machine which keeps the baby in an environment of proper temperature and humidity
Indomethacin   A chemical agent used to close a patent ductus arteriosus
Infusion   Delivery of fluids by a needle or plastic tube; sometimes referred to as a 'drip'
Intravenous feeding   Method of supplying essential nutrients by infusion into a vein
Intraventricular haemorrhage   Bleeding within the ventricular system of the brain
Jaundice   The yellowing of the skin caused by a susbtance produced when red blood cells break down
Mental development   Intellectual growth
Morbidity   A diseased condition or state
Motor development   Growth of the skills that enable a child to move (for example, sit, stand, walk)
Neurologic dysfunction   Disturbance, impairment, or abnormality of the functioning of the nervous system
Oedema   Presence of swelling due to excess fluid in the tissues
Ophthalmologist   A specialist who deals with disorders of the eye
Patent ductus arteriosus   Persistence of communication between the two major arteries coming from the heart — this channel is open during prenatal life, but normally closes shortly after birth
Percentile   A point in a distribution below which falls the percentage of cases indicated by the given percentile, e.g. the tenth percentile denotes the point below which ten per cent of the scores fall
Polyhydramnios   Excessive amount of amniotic fluid
Premature or preterm   A baby born earlier than thirty-seven weeks gestation
Reflux   A backward flow, referring to a type of vomiting or spilling
Respiratory distress syndrome (RDS)   A respiratory condition marked by irregular breathing
Small for gestational age (SGA) or small for dates (SFD)   Low weight for that particular length of pregnancy (usually less than the tenth percentile)
Steroids   A term commonly used to refer to compounds similar to a hormone secreted by the adrenal gland, used to induce maturation of the preterm foetal lung
Term   Thirty-seven to forty-one completed weeks of gestation
Toxaemia   A medical condition or group of conditions, specific to

pregnancy, which includes elevated blood pressure, in association
with oedema (fluid retention) and proteinuria (protein in the urine)
Uterus   Womb
Ventilator   A machine which supports the baby's breathing

Further Reading

Butler, D. and Clay, M. (1979) *Reading Begins at Home* Heinemann Educational Books, Auckland.

Fox, J. (1990) *Bottlefeeding Without Feeling Guilty* Pitman Publishers, Sydney.

Glover, B. (1985) *You and Your Premature Baby* Sheldon Press, United Kingdom.

Green, C. (1990) *Babies — A Parent's Guide to Surviving (and Enjoying!) Baby's First Year* Simon Schuster, Australia.

Goldberg, J. and Taylor, P. (1988) *Premature Infants — Their Continuing Care at Home* Pitman, Sydney.

Gotsch, G. (1990) *Breastfeeding Your Premature Baby* La Leche League International Inc., USA.

Kitchen, W.H., Ryan, M.M., Rickards, A.L. and Lissenden, J.V. (1983) *Premature Babies. A Guide For Parents* Hill of Content Publishing Co. Ltd, Melbourne.

Kitzinger, S. (1989) *Breastfeeding Your Baby* Doubleday, Sydney.

MacDonald, K. (1985) *The Sleep Book* Heinemann Reed, Auckland.

Nance, S. (1982) *Premature Babies: A Handbook for Parents* Arbor House, New York.

Redshaw, M., Rivers, R. and Rosenblatt, D. (1985) *Born Too Early. Special Care For Your Preterm Baby* Oxford University Press, Oxford.

Sammons, W.A.H. and Lewis, J.M. (1985) *Premature Babies. A Different Beginning* C.V. Mosby, St Louis.

Schickedanz, J.A. (1986) *More Than the ABCs. The Early Stages of Reading and Writing.* National Association for the Education of Young Children, Washington DC.

Sears, W. (1987) *Creative Parenting* Collins Dove, Melbourne.

Seymour, F. (1987) *Good Behaviour* GP Books, New Zealand.

Helpful Addresses

Australia

Australian Early Childhood Association Inc.,
Knox Street, Watson ACT 2602, Canberra. Telephone: 06 241 6900.

Childbirth and Parenting Association of Victoria,
49 Taylors Road, Croydon, Melbourne. Telephone: 03 725 4832 and 03 725 3485.

Nursing Mothers' Association of Australia, National Headquarters,
5 Glendale St, Nunawading, Victoria 3131. Telephone: 03 877 5011.

Preterm Infants' Parents' Association,
9 Heathfield St, Eight Mile Plains, Queensland 4123.

New Zealand

Allergy Awareness Association,
PO Box 12-701, Penrose, Auckland 6.

Bereaved Parents,
PO Box 9407, Newmarket, Auckland.

Children in Hospital Liaison Group,
PO Box 10199, Balmoral, Auckland 3.

La Leche League New Zealand,
PO Box 13383, Johnsonville, Wellington.

La Leche League Auckland,
Telephone: 09 846 0752.

Leslie Centre for Family Counselling,
PO Box 74-157, Market Rd, Auckland. Telephone: 09 524 4272.

Multiple Birth Association, PO Box 1258, Wellington. Auckland contact: Carrie Boyd. Telephone: 09 818 3674.

Parent Care National Womens Support Group for Parents of Premature and High Risk Infants,
PO Box 8297, Symonds St, Auckland. Telephone: 09 638 9919.

Parents for Language Disordered Children,
34 Stanley Point Rd, Devonport, Auckland. Telephone: 09 452 386.

Parent Support Groups are associated with the Intensive Care Units of the following: Christchurch Women's Hospital, Christchurch; Grey Hospital, Greymouth; Hutt Hospital, Lower Hutt; Kew Hospital, Invercargill; Memorial Hospital, Hastings; Masterton

Hospital, Masterton; Middlemore Hospital, Auckland; Nelson Hospital, Nelson; Northland Base Hospital, Whangarei; Palmerston North Hospital, Palmerston North; Queen Mary Hospital, Dunedin; Taranaki Base Hospital, New Plymouth; Timaru Hospital, Timaru; Waikato Hospital, Hamilton; Wairau Hospital, Blenheim; Wanganui Hospital, Wanganui; Wellington Women's Hospital, Wellington; Whakatane Hospital, Whakatane; the Special Care Nursery, Tauranga Maternity Annex, Tauranga; the Te Puke Family Unit, Leniham House, Leniham Drive, Te Puke; and c/- Lesley Fisher, Strathallan Station, RD 1, Gisborne.

North America
Association for Childhood Education International,
11141 Georgia Avenue, Wheaton, Washington DC. Telephone: 301 942 2443.
La Leche League International Inc.,
9616 Minneapolis Avenue, Franklin Park, Illinois 60131. Telephone: 708 455 7730.
National Association for the Education of Young Children,
1834 Connecticut Ave, N.W. Washington DC 20009. Telephone: 202 232 8777 or 800 424 2460.
National Institute of Health — Child Health and Human Development, 9000 Rockville Pike, Bethesda. Telephone: 301 496 4000.
Parent Care Inc.,
9041 Colgate St, Indianapolis, Indiana 46268. Telephone: 317 872 9913.
Parent Care,
University of Utah Medical Centre, 50 North Medical Drive, Room 2A210, Salt Lake City, Utah 8413A.
United States Government Health and Human Services — Maternal and Child Health. Telephone: 301 443 2170.

United Kingdom
ACT (Aid for Children with Tracheostomies),
2 Dorset Way, Billericay, Essex CM12 OUD. Telephone: 0277 654425.
Action for Sick Children (formerly NAWCH), (National Association for the Welfare of Children in Hospital),
Argyle House, 29–31 Euston Road, London, NW1 2SD, Telephone: 071 833 2041.

Association of Breastfeeding Mothers (ABM),
  Sydenham Green Health Centre, Holmshaw Close, Sydenham, London, SE 26 4TH. Telephone: 081 778 4769 (telephone recording of breastfeeding counsellors).
BLISS (Baby Life Support Systems),
  17–21 Emerald Street, Holborn, London, W.C.1. Telephone: 071 831 8996.
Caesarean Support Network,
  C/- Yvonne Williams, 55 Cooil Drive, Douglas, Isle of Man. Telephone: 0624 620647.
CAPT (Child Accident Prevention Trust),
  28 Portland Place, London, W1N 4 DE. Telephone: 071 636 2545.
Compassionate Friends,
  6 Denmark Street, Bristol BS1 5DQ. Telephone: 0272 292778.
Contact-a-Family (an umbrella group for families whose children have special needs),
  16 Strutton Ground, London, SW1P 2HP. Telephone: 071 222 2695.
CRY-SIS (Support group for parents of crying infants/children),
  6 Green Lane, Hersham, Walton-on-Thames, Surrey. Telephone: 0932 231149.
Exploring Parenthood,
  Latimer Education Centre, 194 Freston Road, London, W10 6TT. Telephone: 081 960 1678.
Family Planning Association,
  27 Mortimer Street, London, W1. Telephone: 071 636 7866.
La Leche League of Great Britain,
  PO Box B.M., London, WC1N 3XX. Telephone: 071 242 1278.
Maternity Alliance,
  15 Britannia Street, London, WC1. Telephone: 071 837 1265.
Meet-a-Mum Association,
  58 Malden Avenue, South Norwood, London, SE25 4HS. Telephone: 081 656 7318.
National Childbirth Trust (NCT),
  Alexandra House, Oldham Terrace, Acton, London, W3 6NH. Telephone: 081 992 8637.
NIPPERS (National Information for Parents of Prematures: Education, Resources, and Support) (includes bereavement, special needs, and chronic lung disease sub-groups).
  The Sam Segal Perinatal Unit, St Mary's Hospital, London, W2 1NY. Telephone: 071 725 1487.

NIPPERS (*continued*)
   PO Box 1553, Wedmore, Somerset BS28 4LZ. Telephone: 0934 733123.
SANDS (The Stillbirth and Neonatal Death Society),
   28 Portland Place, London, W1N 4DE. Telephone: 071 436 5881.
TAMBA (Twins and Multiple Births Association),
   PO Box 30, Little Sutton, L66 1TH. Telephone: 051 348 0020.
TOPSI (Toxaemia of Pregnancy: Support and Information),
   C/- Laura Kostois, Queen Charlotte's Hospital, Goldhawk Road, London, W6. Telephone: 071 371 8768.

Index